The Definitive Air Fryer Cooking Guide

A Complete Collection of Meat Recipes to Start Your Air Fryer and Boost Your Taste

I0146054

Eva Sheppard

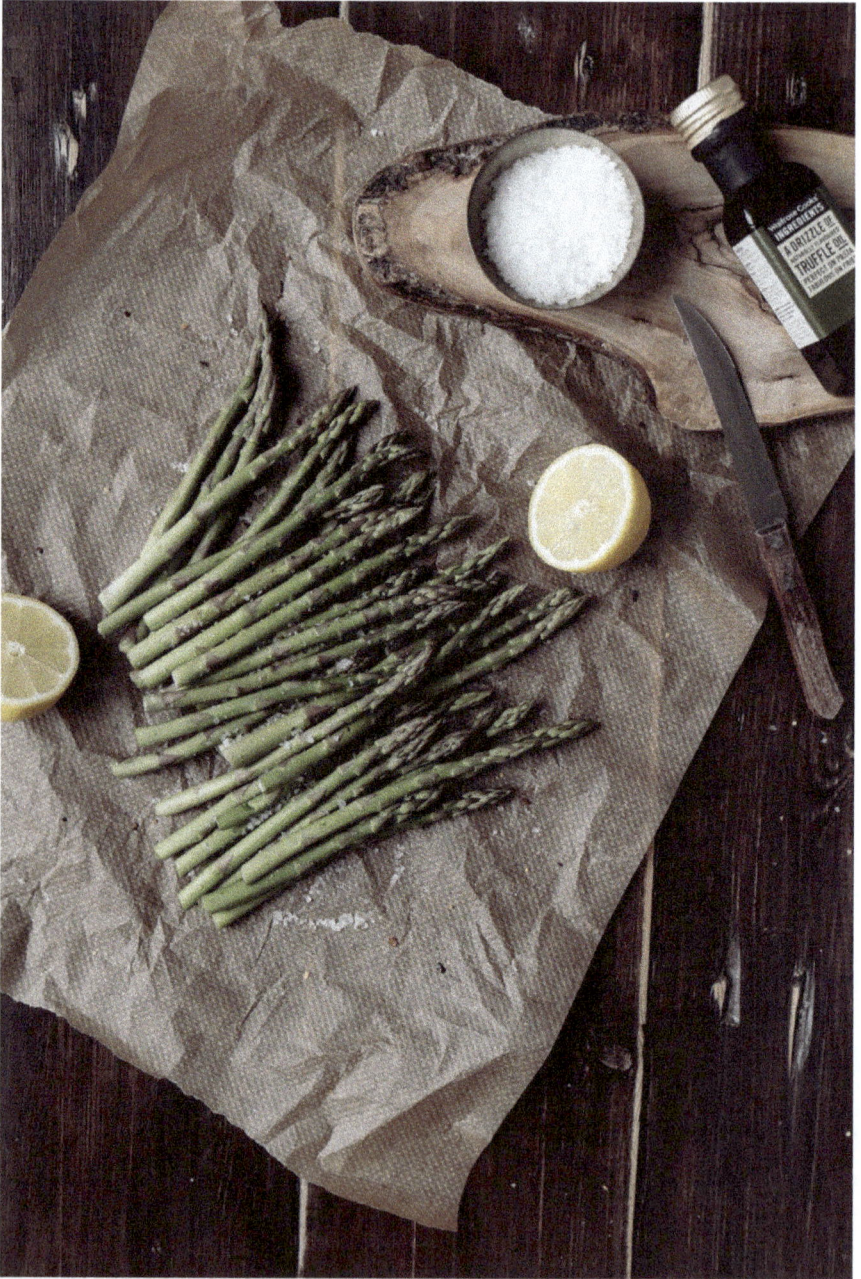

not engaging in the rendering of legal, financial, medical or professional advice. The content within this book has been derived from various sources. Please consult a licensed professional before attempting any techniques outlined in this book.

By reading this document, the reader agrees that under no circumstances is the author responsible for any losses, direct or indirect, which are incurred as a result of the use of information contained within this document, including, but not limited to, — errors, omissions, or inaccuracies.

TABLE OF CONTENT

Nutty Pumpkin with Blue Cheese

Preparation Time: 30 min / Serve: 1

Nutrition Values: Calories: 495; Carbs: 29g; Fat: 27g; Protein: 9g

Ingredients

- ½ small pumpkin
- 2 oz blue cheese , cubed
- 2 tbsp pine nuts
- 1 tbsp olive oil
- ½ cup baby spinach, packed
- 1 spring onion, sliced
- 1 radish, thinly sliced
- 1 tsp vinegar

Directions

1. Preheat the Air fryer to 330 F, and place the pine nuts in a baking dish to toast them for 5 minutes; set aside. Peel the pumpkin and chop it into small pieces. Place in the baking

dish and toss with the olive oil. Increase the temperature to 390 F and cook the pumpkin for 20 minutes.

2. Place the pumpkin in a serving bowl. Add baby spinach, radish and spring onion; toss with the vinegar. Stir in the cubed blue cheese and top with the toasted pine nuts, to serve.

Chili Bean Burritos

Preparation Time: 30 min

Servings: 6

Nutrition Values: Calories: 248; Carbs: 25g; Fat: 8.7g; Protein: 9g

Ingredients

- 6 tortillas
- 1 cup grated cheddar cheese
- 1 can -8 ozbeans
- 1 tsp seasoning, any kind

Directions

1. Preheat the Air fryer to 350 F, and mix the beans with the seasoning. Divide the bean mixture between the tortillas and top with cheddar cheese. Roll the burritos and arrange them on a lined baking dish.

2. Place in the Air fryer and cook for 5 minutes, or to your liking.

Veggie Meatballs

Preparation Time: 30 min

Servings: 3

Nutrition Values: Calories: 288; Carbs: 32g; Fat: 21g; Protein: 6g

Ingredients

- 2 tbsp olive oil
- 2 tbsp soy sauce
- 1 tbsp flax meal
- 2 cups cooked chickpeas
- ½ cup sweet onion, diced
- ½ cup grated carrots
- ½ cup roasted cashews
- Juice of 1 lemon
- ½ tsp turmeric
- 1 tsp cumin
- 1 tsp garlic powder
- 1 cup rolled oats

Directions

1. Combine the oil, onions, and carrots into a baking dish and cook them in the air fryer for 6 minutes at 350 F.

2. Meanwhile, ground the oats and cashews in a food processor. Place them in a large bowl. Process the chickpeas with the lemon juice and soy sauce, until smooth. Add them to the bowl as well.

3. Add onions and carrots to the bowl with chickpeas. Stir in the remaining ingredients; mix until fully incorporated. Make meatballs out of the mixture. Increase the temperature to 370 degrees F and cook for 12 minutes.

Eggplant Cheeseburger

Preparation Time: 10 min / Serve: 1

Nutrition Values: Calories: 399: Carbs: 21g; Fat: 17g; Protein: 8g

Ingredients

- 1 hamburger bun
- 2-inch eggplant slice, cut along the round axis
- 1 mozzarella slice
- 1 red onion cut into 3 rings
- 1 lettuce leaf
- ½ tbsp tomato sauce
- 1 pickle, sliced

Directions

1. Preheat the air fryer to 330 F, and place the eggplant slice to roast for 6 minutes. Place the mozzarella slice on top of the eggplant and cook for 30 more seconds. Spread the tomato sauce on one half of the bun.

2. Place the lettuce leaf on top of the sauce. Place the cheesy eggplant on top of the lettuce. Top with onion rings and pickles, and then with the other bun half and enjoy.

Cheesy Broccoli with Eggs

Preparation Time: 15 min

Servings: 4

Nutrition Values: Calories: 265: Carbs: 19g; Fat: 23g; Protein: 26g

Ingredients

- 1 lb broccoli
- 4 eggs
- 1 cup cheese , shredded
- 1 cup cream
- 1 pinch nutmeg
- 1 tsp ginger powder
- salt and pepper to taste

Directions

1. Steam the broccoli for 5 minutes. Then drain them and add 1 egg, cream, nutmeg, ginger, salt and pepper. Butter small ramekins and spread the mixture. Sprinkle the shredded cheese on top. Cook for 10 minutes at 280 F.

Air-Fried Sweet Potato

Preparation Time: 30min

Servings: 4

Nutrition Values: Calories: 111; Carbs: 12.3g; Fat: 3.8g; Protein: 8.9g

Ingredients

- ½ tsp salt
- ½ tsp garlic powder
- ½ tsp cayenne pepper
- ¼ tsp cumin
- 3 tbsp olive oil
- 3 sweet potatoes, cut into ½-inch thick wedges
- A handful of chopped fresh parsley
- Sea salt

Directions

1. In a bowl, mix salt, garlic powder, chili powder, and cumin. Whisk in oil, and coat the potatoes. Arrange in the Air fryer, without overcrowding, and cook for 20

minutes at 380 F; toss regularly to get the crispy on all sides. Sprinkle with parsley and sea salt, and serve!

Crunchy Parmesan Zucchini

Preparation Time: 40 min

Servings: 4

Nutrition Values: Calories: 369: Carbs: 14g; Fat: 12g; Protein: 9.5g

Ingredients

- 4 small zucchini cut lengthwise
- ½ cup grated Parmesan cheese
- ½ cup breadcrumbs
- ¼ cup melted butter
- ¼ cup chopped parsley
- 4 garlic cloves, minced
- Salt and pepper, to taste

Directions

2. Preheat the Air fryer to 350 F, and in a bowl, mix the breadcrumbs, Parmesan, garlic, and parsley. Season with salt and

pepper, to taste; stir in the melted butter. Arrange the zucchinis with the cut side up.

3. Spread the mixture onto the zucchini evenly. Place half of the zucchinis in the air fryer and cook for 13 minutes.

4. Increase the temperature to 370 F, and cook for 3 more minutes for extra crunchiness. Repeat, and serve hot.

Spinach and Feta Crescent Triangles

Preparation Time: 20 min

Servings: 4

Nutrition Values: Calories: 178; Carbs: 10.8g; Fat: 11.9g; Protein: 8g

Ingredients

- 14 oz store-bought crescent dough
- 1 cup steamed spinach
- 1 cup crumbled feta cheese
- ¼ tsp garlic powder
- 1 tsp chopped oregano
- ¼ tsp salt

Directions

1. Preheat the Air fryer to 350 F, and roll the dough onto a lightly floured flat surface. Combine the feta, spinach, oregano, salt, and garlic powder together in a bowl. Cut the dough into 4 equal pieces.

2. Divide the spinach/feta mixture between the dough pieces. Make sure to place the filling in the center. Fold the dough and secure with a fork. Place onto a lined baking dish, and then in the Air fryer. Cook for 12 minutes, until lightly browned.

Feta Cheese Triangles

Preparation Time: 20 min

Servings: 4

Nutrition Values: Calories: 254; Carbs: 21g; Fat: 19g; Protein: 21g

Ingredients

- 4 oz feta cheese
- 2 sheets filo pastry
- 1 egg yolk
- 2 tbsp parsley, finely chopped
- 1 scallion, finely chopped
- 2 tbsp olive oil
- salt and black pepper

Directions

1. In a large bowl, beat the yolk and mix with the cheese, the chopped parsley and scallion. Season with salt and black pepper. Cut each filo sheet in three parts or strips. Put a teaspoon of the feta mixture on the bottom.

2. Roll the strip in a spinning spiral way until the filling of the inside mixture is completely wrapped in a triangle. Preheat the Air Fryer to 360 F, and brush the surface of the filo with oil. Place up to 5 triangles in the Air frier's basket and cook for 5 minutes. Lower the temperature to 330 F, cook for 3 more minutes or until golden brown.

Eggplant Caviar

Preparation Time: 20 min

Servings: 3

Nutrition Values: Calories: 125; Carbs: 12g; Fat: 3g; Protein: 2g

Ingredients

- 3 medium eggplants
- ½ red onion, chopped and blended
- 2 tbsp balsamic vinegar
- 1 tbsp olive oil
- salt

Directions

1. Arrange the eggplants in the basket and cook them for 15 minutes at 380 F. Remove them and let them cool. Then cut the eggplants in half, lengthwise, and empty their insides with a spoon.

2. Blend the onion in a blender. Put the inside of the eggplants in the blender and process everything. Add the vinegar, olive oil and

salt, then blend again. Serve cool with bread and tomato sauce or ketchup.

Spinach Pie

Preparation time: 10 minutes

Cooking time: 15 minutes

Servings: 4

Ingredients:

- 7 ounces flour
- 2 tablespoons butter
- 7ounces spinach
- 1 tablespoon olive oil
- 2 eggs
- 2 tablespoons milk
- 3 ounces cottage cheese
- Salt and black pepper to the taste
- 1 yellow onion, chopped

Directions:

1. In your food processor, mix flour with butter, 1 egg, milk, salt and pepper, blend well, transfer to a bowl, knead, cover and leave for 10 minutes.

2. Heat up a pan with the oil over medium high heat, add onion and spinach, stir and cook for 2 minutes.

3. Add salt, pepper, the remaining egg and cottage cheese, stir well and take off heat.

4. Divide dough in 4 pieces, roll each piece, place on the bottom of a ramekin, add spinach filling over dough, place ramekins in your air fryer's basket and cook at 360 degrees F for 15 minutes.

5. Serve warm,

6. Enjoy!

Nutrition Values: calories 250, fat 12, fiber 2, carbs 23, protein 12

Balsamic Artichokes

Preparation time: 10 minutes

Cooking time: 7 minutes

Servings: 4

Ingredients:

- 4 big artichokes, trimmed
- Salt and black pepper to the taste
- 2 tablespoons lemon juice
- ¼ cup extra virgin olive oil
- 2 teaspoons balsamic vinegar
- 1 teaspoon oregano, dried
- 2 garlic cloves, minced

Directions:

1. Season artichokes with salt and pepper, rub them with half of the oil and half of the lemon juice, put them in your air fryer and cook at 360 degrees F for 7 minutes.

2. Meanwhile, in a bowl, mix the rest of the lemon juice with vinegar, the remaining oil,

salt, pepper, garlic and oregano and stir very well.

3. Arrange artichokes on a platter, drizzle the balsamic vinaigrette over them and serve.

4. Enjoy!

Nutrition Values: calories 200, fat 3, fiber 6, carbs 12, protein 4

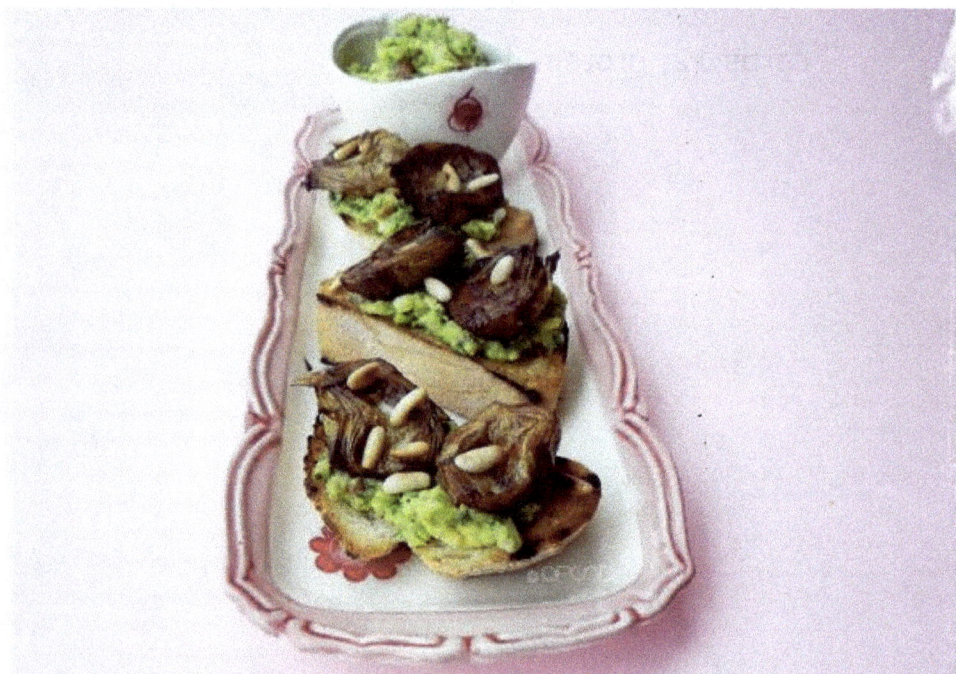

Cheesy Artichokes

Preparation time: 10 minutes

Cooking time: 6 minutes

Servings: 6

Ingredients:

- 14 ounces canned artichoke hearts
- 8 ounces cream cheese
- 16 ounces parmesan cheese, grated
- 10 ounces spinach
- ½ cup chicken stock
- 8 ounces mozzarella, shredded
- ½ cup sour cream
- 3 garlic cloves, minced
- ½ cup mayonnaise
- 1 teaspoon onion powder

Directions:

1. In a pan that fits your air fryer, mix artichokes with stock, garlic, spinach, cream cheese, sour cream, onion powder

and mayo, toss, introduce in your air fryer and cook at 350 degrees F for 6 minutes.

2. Add mozzarella and parmesan, stir well and serve.

3. Enjoy!

Nutrition Values: calories 261, fat 12, fiber 2, carbs 12, protein 15

Artichokes and Special Sauce

Preparation time: 10 minutes

Cooking time: 6 minutes

Servings: 2

Ingredients:

- 2 artichokes, trimmed
- A drizzle of olive oil
- 2 garlic cloves, minced
- 1 tablespoon lemon juice
- For the sauce:
- ¼ cup coconut oil
- ¼ cup extra virgin olive oil
- 3 anchovy fillets
- 3 garlic cloves

Directions:

1. In a bowl, mix artichokes with oil, 2 garlic cloves and lemon juice, toss well, transfer

to your air fryer, cook at 350 degrees F for 6 minutes and divide among plates.

2. In your food processor, mix coconut oil with anchovy, 3 garlic cloves and olive oil, blend very well, drizzle over artichokes and serve.

3. Enjoy!

Nutrition Values: calories 261, fat 4, fiber 7, carbs 20, protein 12

Beet Salad and Parsley Dressing

Preparation time: 10 minutes

Cooking time: 14 minutes

Servings: 4

Ingredients:

- 4 beets
- 2 tablespoons balsamic vinegar
- A bunch of parsley, chopped
- Salt and black pepper to the taste
- 1 tablespoon extra virgin olive oil
- 1 garlic clove, chopped
- 2 tablespoons capers

Directions:

1. Put beets in your air fryer and cook them at 360 degrees F for 14 minutes.

2. Meanwhile, in a bowl, mix parsley with garlic, salt, pepper, olive oil and capers and stir very well.

3. Transfer beets to a cutting board, leave them to cool down, peel them, slice put them in a salad bowl.

4. Add vinegar, drizzle the parsley dressing all over and serve.

5. Enjoy!

Nutrition Values: calories 70, fat 2, fiber 1, carbs 6, protein 4

Beets and Blue Cheese Salad

Preparation time: 10 minutes

Cooking time: 14 minutes

Servings: 6

Ingredients:

- 6 beets, peeled and quartered
- Salt and black pepper to the taste
- ¼ cup blue cheese, crumbled
- 1 tablespoon olive oil

Directions:

1. Put beets in your air fryer, cook them at 350 degrees F for 14 minutes and transfer them to a bowl.

2. Add blue cheese, salt, pepper and oil, toss and serve.

3. Enjoy!

Nutrition Values: calories 100, fat 4, fiber 4, carbs 10, protein 5

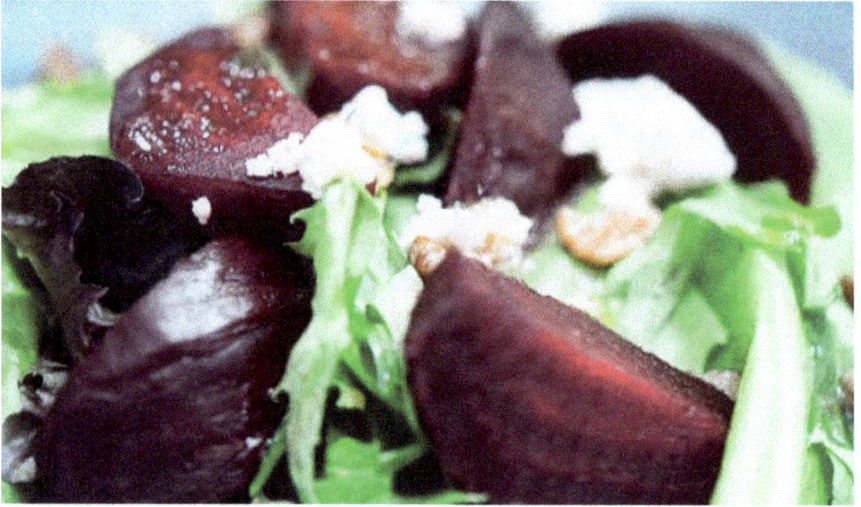

Beets and Arugula Salad

Preparation time: 10 minutes

Cooking time: 10 minutes

Servings: 4

Ingredients:

- 1 and ½ pounds beets, peeled and quartered
- A drizzle of olive oil
- 2 teaspoons orange zest, grated
- 2 tablespoons cider vinegar
- ½ cup orange juice
- 2 tablespoons brown sugar
- 2 scallions, chopped
- 2 teaspoons mustard
- 2 cups arugula

Directions:

1. Rub beets with the oil and orange juice, place them in your air fryer and cook at 350 degrees F for 10 minutes.

2. Transfer beet quarters to a bowl, add scallions, arugula and orange zest and toss.

3. In a separate bowl, mix sugar with mustard and vinegar, whisk well, add to salad, toss and serve.

4. Enjoy!

Nutrition Values: calories 121, fat 2, fiber 3, carbs 11, protein 4

Beet, Tomato and Goat Cheese Mix

Preparation time: 30 minutes

Cooking time: 14 minutes

Servings: 8

Ingredients:

- 8 small beets, trimmed, peeled and halved
- 1 red onion, sliced
- 4 ounces goat cheese, crumbled
- 1 tablespoon balsamic vinegar
- Salt and black pepper to the taste
- 2 tablespoons sugar
- 1 pint mixed cherry tomatoes, halved
- 2 ounces pecans
- 2 tablespoons olive oil

Directions:

1. Put beets in your air fryer, season them with salt and pepper, cook at 350 degrees

F for 14 minutes and transfer to a salad bowl.

2. Add onion, cherry tomatoes and pecans and toss.

3. In another bowl, mix vinegar with sugar and oil, whisk well until sugar dissolves and add to salad.

4. Also add goat cheese, toss and serve.

5. Enjoy!

Nutrition Values: calories 124, fat 7, fiber 5, carbs 12, protein 6

Broccoli Salad

Preparation time: 10 minutes

Cooking time: 8 minutes

Servings: 4

Ingredients:

- 1 broccoli head, florets separated
- 1 tablespoon peanut oil
- 6 garlic cloves, minced
- 1 tablespoon Chinese rice wine vinegar
- Salt and black pepper to the taste

Directions:

1. In a bowl, mix broccoli with salt, pepper and half of the oil, toss, transfer to your air fryer and cook at 350 degrees F for 8 minutes, shaking the fryer halfway.

2. Transfer broccoli to a salad bowl, add the rest of the peanut oil, garlic and rice vinegar, toss really well and serve.

3. Enjoy!

Nutrition Values: calories 121, fat 3, fiber 4, carbs 4, protein 4

Brussels Sprouts and Tomatoes Mix

Preparation time: 5 minutes

Cooking time: 10 minutes

Servings: 4

Ingredients:

- 1 pound Brussels sprouts, trimmed
- Salt and black pepper to the taste
- 6 cherry tomatoes, halved
- ¼ cup green onions, chopped
- 1 tablespoon olive oil

Directions:

1. Season Brussels sprouts with salt and pepper, put them in your air fryer and cook at 350 degrees F for 10 minutes.

2. Transfer them to a bowl, add salt, pepper, cherry tomatoes, green onions and olive oil, toss well and serve.

3. Enjoy!

Nutrition Values: calories 121, fat 4, fiber 4, carbs 11, protein 4

Artichokes and Mayonnaise Mix with Parmesan

Preparation Time: 20 minutes

Servings: 6

Ingredients:

- canned artichoke hearts - 14 ounces
- A drizzle of olive oil
- parmesan cheese - 16 ounces, grated
- garlic cloves - 3, minced
- mayonnaise - ½ cup
- garlic powder - 1 teaspoon

Directions:

1. Pour the artichokes with the oil, garlic, and garlic powder in a pan that fits right into your fryer, mix properly and toss well.

2. Put the pan in the fryer and cook at a temperature of 350 o F for 15 minutes.

3. Let the mix cool down, then add the mayo, and toss well to coat.

4. Cut into different plates, then sprinkle the parmesan on top, and serve right away.

Nutrition Values:

calories 200, fat 11, fiber 3, carbs 9, protein 4

Coconut Artichokes Recipe

Preparation Time: 20 minutes

Servings: 2

Ingredients:

- Artichokes - 2, washed, trimmed and halved
- garlic cloves - 2, minced
- Coconut - ¼ cup, shredded
- Lemon Juice - 1
- coconut oil - 1 tablespoon, melted

Directions:

1. Mix the artichokes with the garlic, oil, and lemon juice in a bowl; and toss well to ensure it is well coated.

2. Transfer them artichokes to the air fryer and cook at a temperature of 360 o F. Do this for 15 minutes.

3. Cut the artichokes into different plates, then sprinkle the coconut as toppings, and serve.

4. Enjoy your meal!

Nutrition Values:

calories 213, fat 8, fiber 6, carbs 13, protein 6

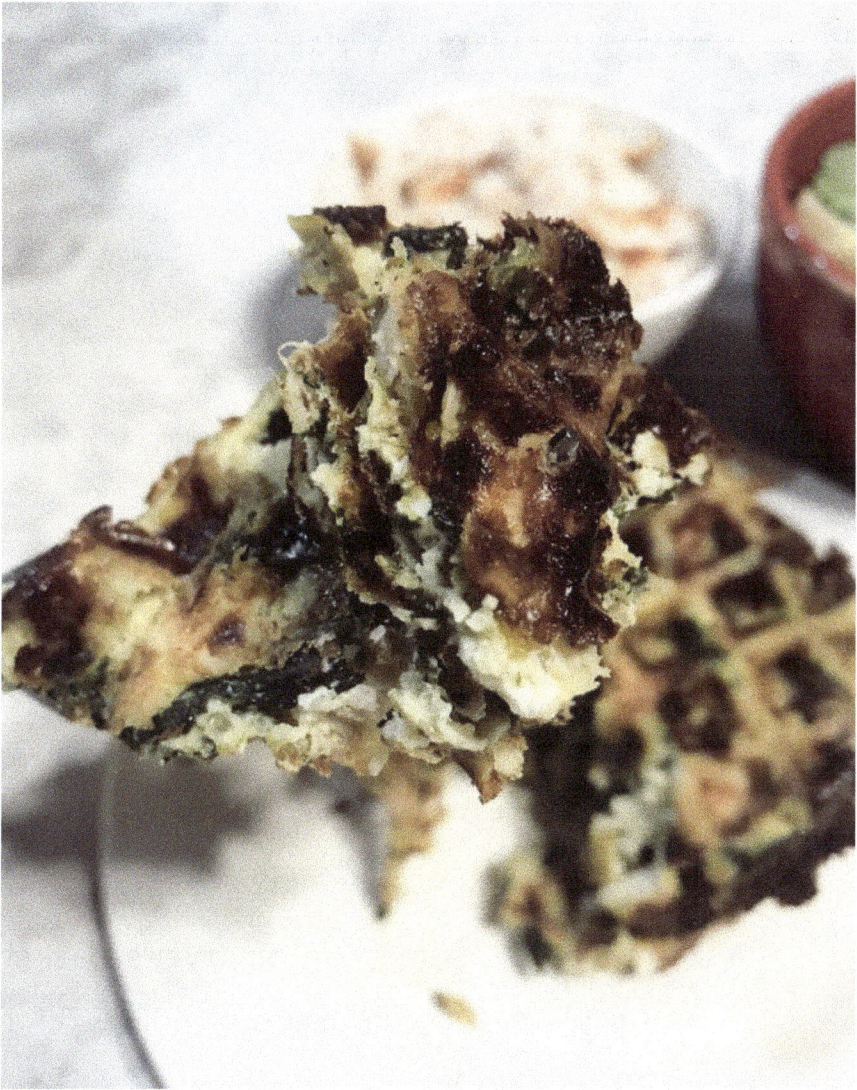

Seasoned Wrapped Asparagus Recipe

Preparation Time: 10 minutes

Servings: 4

Ingredients:

- asparagus spears - 8, trimmed
- prosciutto slices - 8 ounces
- A pinch of salt and black pepper

Directions:

1. First, wrap the asparagus with slices of prosciutto; then add salt and pepper to taste.

2. Introduce all of it to an air fryer's basket and cook at a temperature of 400 o F for about 5 minutes.

3. Cut into different plates and serve.

Nutrition Values:

calories 100, fat 2, fiber 5, carbs 8, protein 4

Preparation Time: 10 minutes

Servings: 4

Ingredients:

- extra virgin olive oil - 1 teaspoon
- asparagus - 1 bunch, trimmed
- Cajun seasoning - ½ tablespoon

Directions:

1. Mix the asparagus with the oil and Cajun seasoning in a clean bowl; coat the asparagus properly.

2. Move the asparagus to your air fryer and cook at a temperature of 400 o F for about 5 minutes.

3. Cut all of it into different plates and serve.

Nutrition Values:

calories 151, fat 3, fiber 4, carbs 9, protein 4

Seasoned Squash Salad

Preparation Time: 17 minutes

Servings: 4

Ingredients:

- butternut squash - 1, cubed
- balsamic vinegar - 2 tablespoons
- cilantro - 1 bunch, chopped
- Salt and black pepper to taste
- olive oil - 1 tablespoon

Directions:

1. Place the squash in the air fryer, then sprinkle a pinch of salt and pepper to taste. Add oil to the mix and toss well to coat.

2. Cook at a temperature of 400 o F for about 15 minutes.

3. Move the squash to a clean bowl, before adding the vinegar and cilantro. Toss the mix well.

4. Serve away and enjoy your meal!

Nutrition Values:

calories 151, fat 4, fiber 7, carbs 11, protein 8

Balsamic Asparagus

Preparation time: 5 minutes

Cooking time: 5 minutes

Servings: 4

Ingredients:

- 1 asparagus bunch, trimmed and halved
- Salt and black pepper to taste
- 2 tablespoons lime juice
- 2 tablespoons olive oil
- 2 teaspoons balsamic vinegar
- 1 teaspoon oregano, dried

Directions:

1. In a bowl, combine all ingredients and toss.

2. Put the asparagus in your air fryer's basket and cook at 400 degrees F for 5 minutes.

3. Divide the asparagus between plates and serve.

Nutrition Values: calories 190, fat 3, fiber 6, carbs 8, protein 4

Cheesy Asparagus

Preparation time: 5 minutes

Cooking time: 6 minutes

Servings: 6

Ingredients:

- 14 ounces asparagus, trimmed
- 8 ounces cream cheese, softened
- 16 ounces cheddar cheese, grated
- ½ cup sour cream
- 3 garlic cloves, minced
- 1 teaspoon garlic powder

Directions:

1. In a pan that fits your air fryer, the mix asparagus with the cream cheese, sour cream, garlic powder, and garlic; toss.

2. Sprinkle the cheddar cheese on top, and then place the pan in the fryer.

3. Cook at 400 degrees F for 6 minutes.

4. Divide between plates and serve.

Nutrition Values: calories 191, fat 8, fiber 2, carbs 12, protein 8

Simple Fennel Mix

Preparation time: 10 minutes

Cooking time: 12 minutes

Servings: 2

Ingredients:

- 2 fennel bulbs, trimmed and halved

- A drizzle of olive oil

- 2 garlic cloves, minced

- 1 tablespoon lime juice

- 1 teaspoon sweet paprika

Directions:

1. In a bowl, combine all ingredients and toss.

2. Put the fennel in your air fryer's basket and cook at 400 degrees F for 12 minutes.

3. Divide between plates and serve.

Nutrition Values: calories 131, fat 4, fiber 7, carbs 10, protein 8

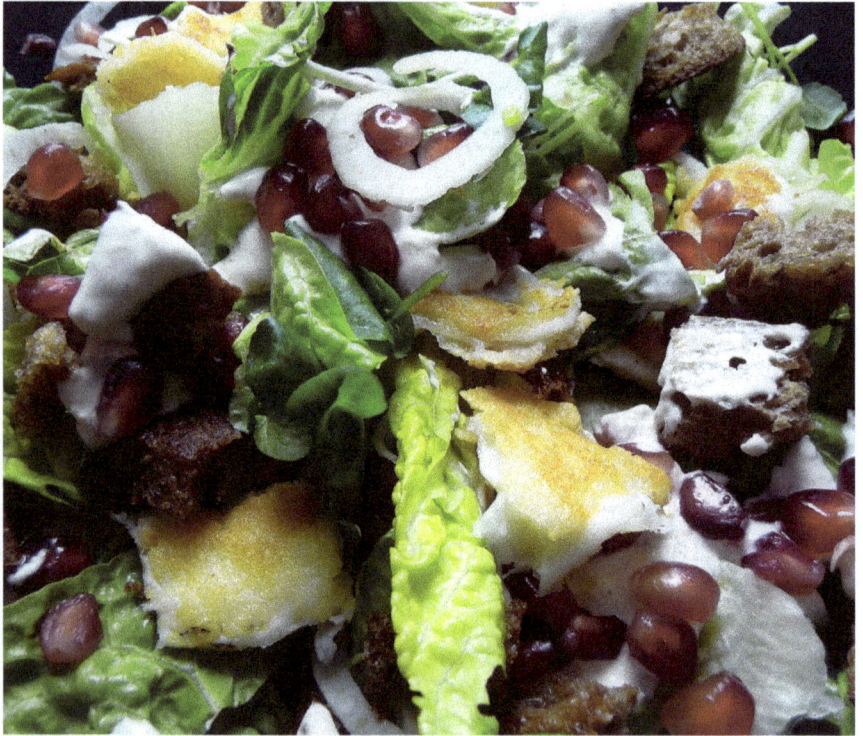

Beets and Capers

Preparation time: 5 minutes

Cooking time: 20 minutes

Servings: 4

Ingredients:

- 4 beets, peeled and cut into wedges
- 2 tablespoons balsamic vinegar
- 1 tablespoon cilantro, chopped
- Salt and black pepper to taste
- 1 tablespoon olive oil
- 2 tablespoons capers

Directions:

1. Put the beet wedges in your air fryer's basket and cook at 400 degrees F for 20 minutes.

2. Transfer the beet wedges to a salad bowl, and then add the remaining ingredients.

3. Toss, serve, and enjoy.

Nutrition Values: calories 70, fat 1, fiber 1, carbs 6, protein 4

Sesame Seed Beets Mix

Preparation time: 10 minutes

Cooking time: 20 minutes

Servings: 6

Ingredients:

- 6 beets, peeled and quartered
- Salt and black pepper to taste
- 1 tablespoon sesame seeds, toasted
- 1 tablespoon red wine vinegar
- 1 tablespoon olive oil

Directions:

1. Put the beets in your air fryer's basket and cook at 400 degrees F for 20 minutes.

2. Transfer the beets to a bowl, and add all remaining ingredients.

3. Toss and serve.

Nutrition Values: calories 100, fat 2, fiber 4, carbs 7, protein 5

Beets and Kale Mix

Preparation time: 5 minutes

Cooking time: 20 minutes

Servings: 4

Ingredients:

- 1½ pounds beets, peeled and quartered
- 1 tablespoon olive oil
- 2 tablespoons balsamic vinegar
- ½ cup orange juice
- Salt and black pepper to taste
- 2 scallions, chopped
- 2 cups kale leaves

Directions:

1. Put the beets in your air fryer's basket and cook at 400 degrees F for 15 minutes.

2. Add the kale leaves and cook for another 5 minutes.

3. Transfer the beets and kale to a bowl and add all remaining ingredients.

4. Toss, serve, and enjoy.

Nutrition Values: calories 151, fat 2, fiber 3, carbs 9, protein 4

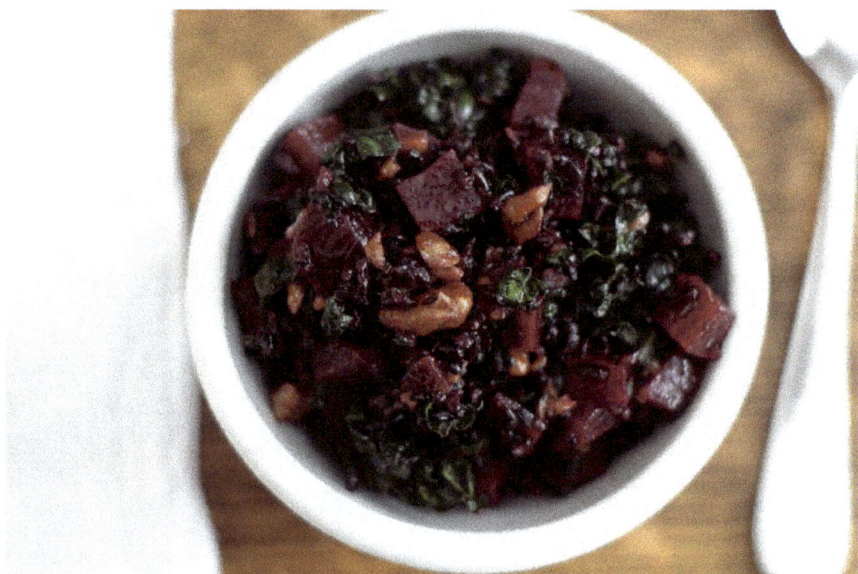

Beet and Tomato Salad

Preparation time: 5 minutes

Cooking time: 25 minutes

Servings: 6

Ingredients:

- 8 small beets, trimmed, peeled and cut into wedges

- 1 red onion, sliced

- 1 tablespoon balsamic vinegar

- Salt and black pepper to taste

- 1 pint mixed cherry tomatoes, halved

- 2 ounces pecans, chopped

- 2 tablespoons olive oil

Directions:

1. Put the beets in your air fryer's basket, and add the salt, pepper, and 1 tablespoon of the oil.

2. Cook at 400 degrees F for 15 minutes.

3. Transfer the beets to a pan that fits your air fryer, and add the onions, tomatoes, pecans, and remaining 1 tablespoon of the oil; toss well.

4. Cook at 400 degrees F for 10 more minutes.

5. Divide between plates and serve.

Nutrition Values: calories 144, fat 7, fiber 5, carbs 8, protein 6

Cauliflower Mix

Preparation time: 5 minutes

Cooking time: 7 minutes

Servings: 4

Ingredients:

- 1 cauliflower head, florets separated

- 1 tablespoon peanut oil

- 6 garlic cloves, minced

- 1 tablespoon Chinese rice wine vinegar

- Salt and black pepper to taste

Directions:

1. Mix all ingredients in a bowl.

2. Put the mixture in the fryer and cook at 400 degrees F for 7 minutes.

3. Divide between plates and serve.

Nutrition Values: calories 141, fat 3, fiber 4, carbs 4, protein 2

Broccoli and Tomatoes

Preparation time: 5 minutes

Cooking time: 7 minutes

Servings: 4

Ingredients:

- 1 broccoli head, florets separated
- Salt and black pepper to taste
- 6 cherry tomatoes, halved
- ¼ cup scallions, chopped
- 1 tablespoon olive oil

Directions:

1. Put the broccoli florets in your air fryer's basket, and add the salt, pepper, and ½ tablespoon of the oil; toss well.

2. Cook at 380 degrees F for 7 minutes.

3. Transfer the broccoli to a bowl, and add the tomatoes, scallions, salt, pepper, and the remaining ½ tablespoon of oil.

4. Toss and serve.

Nutrition Values: calories 111, fat 4, fiber 4, carbs 9, protein 2

Teriyaki Cauliflower

Preparation Time: 20 min

Servings: 4

Nutrition Values: Calories: 147; Carbs: 18.2g; Fat: 7.1g; Protein: 3.4g

Ingredients

- 1 big cauliflower head, cut into florets
- ½ cup soy sauce
- 3 tbsp brown sugar
- 1 tsp sesame oil
- ⅓ cup water
- ½ chili powder
- 2 cloves garlic, chopped
- 1 tsp cornstarch

Directions

1. In a measuring cup, whisk soy sauce, sugar, sesame oil, water, chili powder, garlic and cornstarch, until smooth. In a

bowl, add cauliflower, and pour teriyaki sauce over the top; toss with hands until well-coated.

2. Take the cauliflower to the Air fryer's basket and cook for 14 minutes at 340 F, turning once halfway through. When ready, check if the cauliflower is cooked but not too soft. Serve with rice and edamame beans!

Sweet Potato French Fries

Preparation Time: 30 min

Servings: 4

Nutrition Values: Calories: 176; Carbs: 20.3g; Fat: 10.1g; Protein: 1.6g

Ingredients

- ½ tsp salt
- ½ tsp garlic powder
- ½ tsp chili powder
- ¼ tsp cumin
- 3 tbsp olive oil
- 3 sweet potatoes, cut into thick strips

Directions

1. In a bowl, mix salt, garlic powder, chili powder, and cumin, and whisk in oil. Coat the strips well in this mixture and arrange them in the Air fryer's basket, without overcrowding. Cook for 20 minutes at 380 F, or until crispy.

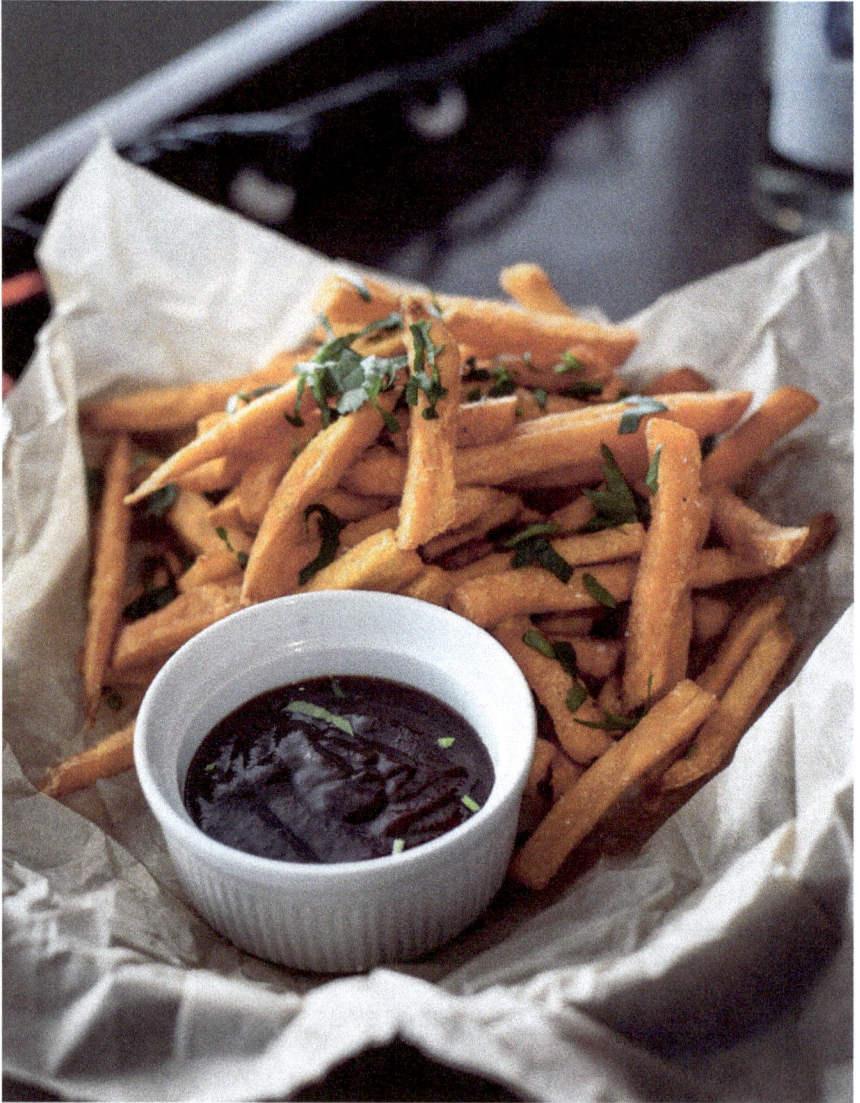

Spicy Mixed Veggie Bites

Preparation Time: 1 hr 30 min

Servings: 13 to 16 bites

Nutrition Values: Calories: 160; Carbs: 3g; Fat: 8g; Protein: 3g

Ingredients

- 1 medium cauliflower, cut in florets
- 6 medium carrots, diced
- 1 medium broccoli, cut in florets
- 1 onion, diced
- ½ cup garden peas
- 2 leeks, sliced thinly
- 1 small zucchini, chopped
- ⅓ cup flour
- 1 tbsp garlic paste
- 2 tbsp olive oil
- 1 tbsp curry paste
- 2 tsp mixed spice
- 1 tsp coriander

- 1 tsp cumin powder

- 1 ½ cups milk

- 1 tsp ginger paste

- Salt and pepper to taste

Directions

1. In a pot, steam all vegetables, except the leek and courgette, for 10 minutes; set aside. Place a wok over medium heat, and add the onion, ginger, garlic and olive oil. Stir-fry until onions turn transparent. Add in leek, zucchini and curry paste. Stir and cook for 5 minutes. Add all spices and milk; stir and simmer for 10 minutes.

2. Once the sauce has reduced, add the steamed veggies; mix evenly. Transfer to a bowl and refrigerate for 1 hour. Remove the veggie base from the fridge and mold into bite sizes. Arrange the veggie bites in the fryer basket and cook at 350 F for 10 minutes. Once ready, serve warm with yogurt sauce.

Brussels Sprouts with Garlic Aioli

Preparation Time: 25 min

Servings: 4

Nutrition Values: Calories: 42; Carbs: 0g; Fat: 2.6g; Protein: 4.9g

Ingredients

- 1 lb brussels sprouts, trimmed and excess leaves removed
- Salt and pepper to taste
- 1 ½ tbsp olive oil
- 2 tsp lemon juice
- 1 tsp powdered chili
- 3 cloves garlic
- ¾ cup mayonnaise, whole egg
- 2 cups water

Directions

1. Place a skillet over medium heat on a stove top, add the garlic cloves with the peels on

it and roast until lightly brown and fragrant. Remove the skillet and place a pot with water over the same heat; bring to a boil.

2. Using a knife, cut the brussels sprouts in halves lengthwise. Add to the boiling water to blanch for just 3 minutes. Drain through a sieve and set aside. Preheat the Air fryer to 350 F. Remove the garlic from the skillet to a plate; peel, crush and set aside. Add olive oil to the skillet and light the fire to medium heat on the stove top.

3. Stir in the brussels sprouts, season with pepper and salt; sauté for 2 minutes and turn off the heat. Pour the brussels sprouts in the fryer's basket and cook for 5 minutes.

4. Meanwhile, make the garlic aioli. In a bowl, add mayonnaise, crushed garlic, lemon juice, powdered chili, pepper and salt; mix well. Remove the brussels sprouts onto a serving bowl and serve with the garlic aioli.

Cheesy Stuffed Peppers

Preparation Time: 40 min

Servings: 4

Nutrition Values: Calories: 115; Carbs: 0g; Fat: 16g; Protein: 13g

Ingredients

- 4 green peppers
- Salt and pepper to taste
- ½ cup olive oil
- 1 red onion, chopped
- 1 large tomato, chopped
- ½ cup crumbled Goat cheese
- 3 cups cauliflower, chopped
- 2 tbsp grated Parmesan cheese
- 2 tbsp chopped basil
- 1 tbsp lemon zest

Directions

1. Preheat the Air Fryer to 350 F, and cut the peppers a quarter way from the head down and lengthwise. Remove the membrane

and seeds. Season the peppers with pepper, salt, and drizzle olive oil over.

2. Place the pepper bottoms in the fryer's basket and cook them for 5 minutes at 350 F to soften a little bit.

3. In a mixing bowl, add the tomatoes, goat cheese, lemon zest, basil, and cauliflower; season with salt and pepper, and mix well. Remove the bottoms from the Air fryer to a flat surface and spoon the cheese mixture into them.

4. Sprinkle Parmesan on top of each and gently place in the basket; cook for 15 minutes. Serve warm.

Cheesy Mushroom and Cauliflower Balls

Preparation Time: 50 min

Servings: 4

Nutrition Values: Calories: 115; Carbs: 4.1g; Fat: 8.6g; Protein: 5.6g

Ingredients

- ½ lb mushrooms, diced
- 3 tbsp olive oil
- 1 small red onion, chopped
- 3 cloves garlic, minced
- 3 cups cauliflower, chopped
- 2 tbsp chicken stock
- 1 cup breadcrumbs
- 1 cup Grana Padano cheese
- ¼ cup coconut oil
- 2 sprigs chopped fresh thyme
- Salt and pepper to taste

Directions

1. Place a skillet over medium heat on a stove top. Add olive oil, once heated, sauté garlic and onion, until translucent.

2. Add the mushrooms, stir-fry for 4 minutes; add the cauliflower and stir-fry for 5 minutes. Pour in the stock, thyme, and simmer until the cauliflower has absorbed the stock. Add Grana Padano cheese, pepper, and salt.

3. Stir and turn off the heat. Allow the mixture cool and make bite-size balls of the mixture. Place them in a plate and refrigerate for 30 minutes to harden. Preheat the Air Fryer to 350 F.

4. In a bowl, add the breadcrumbs and coconut oil and mix well. Remove the mushroom balls from the refrigerator, stir the breadcrumb mixture again, and roll the balls in the breadcrumb mixture.

5. Place the balls in the Air fryer's basket without overcrowding, and cook for 15

minutes, tossing every 5 minutes for an even cook. Repeat until all the mushroom balls are fried. Serve with sautéed zoodles and tomato sauce.

Vegetable Croquettes

Preparation Time: 1 hr 30 min

Servings: 3

Nutrition Values: Calories: 24; Carbs: 2.6g; Fat: 0.3g; Protein: 3.3g

Ingredients

- 1 lb red potatoes
- 2 cups water
- 1 ¼ cups milk
- Salt to taste
- 2 tsp + 3 tsp butter
- 2 tsp olive oil
- 2 red peppers, chopped
- ½ cup baby spinach, chopped
- 3 mushrooms, chopped
- 1/6 broccoli florets, chopped
- 1/6 cup sliced green onion
- ½ red onion, chopped
- 2 cloves garlic, minced

- 1 medium carrot, grated

- ⅓ cup flour

- 2 tbsp cornstarch

- 1 ½ cups breadcrumbs

- Cooking spray

Directions

1. Place the potatoes in a pot, add the water, and bring it to boil over medium heat on a stove top. Boil until tender and mashable. Drain the potatoes through a sieve and place them in a bowl.

2. Add the 2 teaspoons of butter, 1 cup of milk, and salt. Use a potato masher to mash well; set aside.

3. Place a skillet over medium heat on a stove top and melt the remaining butter. Add the onion, garlic, red peppers, broccoli, and mushrooms; stir-fry for 2 minutes. Add green onion and spinach, and cook until the spinach wilts.

4. Season with salt and stir. Turn the heat off and pour the veggie mixture into the potato mash. Use the potato masher to mash the veggies into the potatoes; allow cooling. Using your hands, form oblong balls of the mixture and place them on a baking sheet in a single layer. Refrigerate for 30 minutes.

5. In 3 separate bowls, add breadcrumbs in one, flour in another, and cornstarch, remaining milk and salt in a third bowl. Mix cornstarch, salt and 1 tbsp of water. Remove the patties from the fridge. Preheat the fryer to 390 F.

6. Dredge each veggie mold in flour, then in the cornstarch mixture, and then in the breadcrumbs. Place the patties in batches in a single layer in the basket without overlapping. Spray with olive oil and cook for 2 minutes. Flip, spray them with cooking spray and cook for more 3 minutes.

Remove to a wire rack and serve with tomato sauce.

Curried Cauliflower Florets

Preparation Time: 34 min

Servings: 4

Nutrition Values: Calories: 123; Carbs: 2g; Fat: 11g; Protein: 5g

Ingredients

- 1 large cauliflower head
- Salt to taste
- 1 ½ tbsp curry powder
- ½ cup olive oil
- ⅓ cup fried pine nuts

Directions

1. Preheat the Air Fryer to 390 F, and mix the pine nuts and 1 tsp of olive oil, in a medium bowl. Pour them in the air fryer's basket and cook for 2 minutes; remove to cool.

2. Place the cauliflower on a cutting board. Use a knife to cut them into 1-inch florets. Place them in a large mixing bowl. Add the curry powder, salt, and the remaining olive

oil; mix well. Place the cauliflower florets in the fryer's basket in 2 batches, and cook each batch for 10 minutes. Remove the curried florets onto a serving platter, sprinkle with the pine nuts, and toss. Serve the florets with tomato sauce or as a side to a meat dish.

Roasted Rosemary Squash

Preparation Time: 30 min

Servings: 2

Nutrition Values: Calories: 123; Carbs: 25.7g; Fat: 0.2g; Protein: 1.3g

Ingredients

- 1 butternut squash
- 1 tbsp dried rosemary
- Cooking spray
- Salt to season

Directions

1. Place the butternut squash on a cutting board and peel it; cut it in half and remove the seeds. Cut the pulp into wedges and season with salt.

2. Preheat the Air Fryer to 350 F, spray the squash wedges with cooking spray and sprinkle with rosemary. Grease the fryer's basket with cooking spray and place the wedges inside it without overlapping. Slide

the fryer basket back in and cook for 20 minutes, flipping once halfway through. Serve with maple syrup and goat cheese.

Eggplant Gratin with Mozzarella Crust

Preparation Time: 30 min

Servings: 2 to 3

Nutrition Values: Calories: 317; Carbs: 2g; Fat: 16.83g; Protein: 12g

Ingredients

- 1 cup cubed eggplant
- ¼ cup chopped red pepper
- ¼ cup chopped green pepper
- ¼ cup chopped onion
- ⅓ cup chopped tomatoes
- 1 clove garlic, minced
- 1 tbsp sliced pimiento-stuffed olives
- 1 tsp capers
- ¼ tsp dried basil
- ¼ tsp dried marjoram
- Salt and pepper to taste
- Cooking spray

- ¼ cup grated mozzarella cheese
- 1 tbsp breadcrumbs

Directions

1. Preheat the Air Fryer to 300 F, and in a bowl, add the eggplant, green pepper, red pepper, onion, tomatoes, olives, garlic, basil marjoram, capers, salt, and pepper. Lightly grease a baking dish with the olive oil cooking spray.

2. Ladle the eggplant mixture into the baking dish and level it using the vessel. Sprinkle the mozzarella cheese on top and cover with the breadcrumbs. Place the dish in the Air Fryer and cook for 20 minutes. Serve with rice.

Three Veg Bake

Preparation Time: 30 min

Servings: 3

Nutrition Values: Calories: 50; Carbs: 4g; Fat: 2g; Protein: 2g

Ingredients

- 3 turnips, sliced
- 1 large red onion, cut into rings
- 1 large zucchini, sliced
- Salt and pepper to taste
- 2 cloves garlic, crushed
- 1 bay leaf, cut in 6 pieces
- 1 tbsp olive oil
- Cooking spray

Directions

1. Place the turnips, onion, and zucchini in a bowl. Toss with olive oil and season with salt and pepper.

2. Preheat the Air Fryer to 330 F, and place the veggies into a baking pan that fits in the Air fryer. Slip the bay leaves in the different parts of the slices and tuck the garlic cloves in between the slices.

3. Insert the pan in the Air fryer's basket and cook for 15 minutes. Serve warm with as a side to a meat dish or salad.

Easy Roast Winter Vegetable Delight

Preparation Time: 30 min

Servings: 2

Nutrition Values: Calories: 50; Carbs: 5g; Fat: 3g; Protein: 2g

Ingredients

- 1 parsnip, peeled and sliced in a 2-inch thickness
- 1 cup chopped butternut squash
- 2 small red onions, cut in wedges
- 1 cup chopped celery
- 1 tbsp chopped fresh thyme
- Salt and pepper to taste
- 2 tsp olive oil

Directions

1. Preheat the Air Fryer to 200 F, and in a bowl, add turnip, squash, red onions, celery, thyme, pepper, salt, and olive oil;

mix well. Pour the vegetables into the fryer's basket and cook for 16 minutes, tossing once halfway through.

Potato, Eggplant, and Zucchini Chips

Preparation Time: 45 min

Servings: 4

Nutrition Values: Calories: 120; Carbs: 6g; Fat: 3.5g; Protein: 3g

Ingredients

- 1 large eggplant
- 5 potatoes
- 3 zucchinis
- ½ cup cornstarch
- ½ cup water
- ½ cup olive oil
- Salt to season

Directions

1. Preheat the Air Fryer to 390 F, and cut the eggplant and zucchini in long 3-inch strips. Peel and cut the potatoes into 3-inch strips; set aside. In a bowl, stir in cornstarch,

water, salt, pepper, oil, eggplants, zucchini, and potatoes.

2. Place one-third of the veggie strips in the fryer's basket and cook them for 12 minutes. Once ready, transfer them to a serving platter. Repeat the cooking process for the remaining veggie strips. Serve warm.

Stuffed Mushrooms with bacon & Cheese

Preparation Time: 20 min

Servings: 3 to 4

Nutrition Values: Calories: 67; Carbs: 0.2g; Fat: 3.5g; Protein: 2.7g

Ingredients

- 14 small button mushrooms
- 1 clove garlic, minced
- alt and pepper to taste
- 4 slices bacon, chopped
- ¼ cup grated Cheddar cheese
- 1 tbsp olive oil
- 1 tbsp chopped parsley

Directions

1. Preheat the Air Fryer to 390 F, and in a bowl, add the oil, bacon, cheddar cheese, parsley, salt, pepper, and garlic. Mix well with a spoon. Cut the stalks of the

mushroom off and fill each cap with the bacon mixture.

2. Press the bacon mixture into the caps to avoid from falling off. Place the stuffed mushrooms in the fryer's basket and cook at 390 F for 8 minutes. Once golden and crispy, plate them and serve with a green salad.

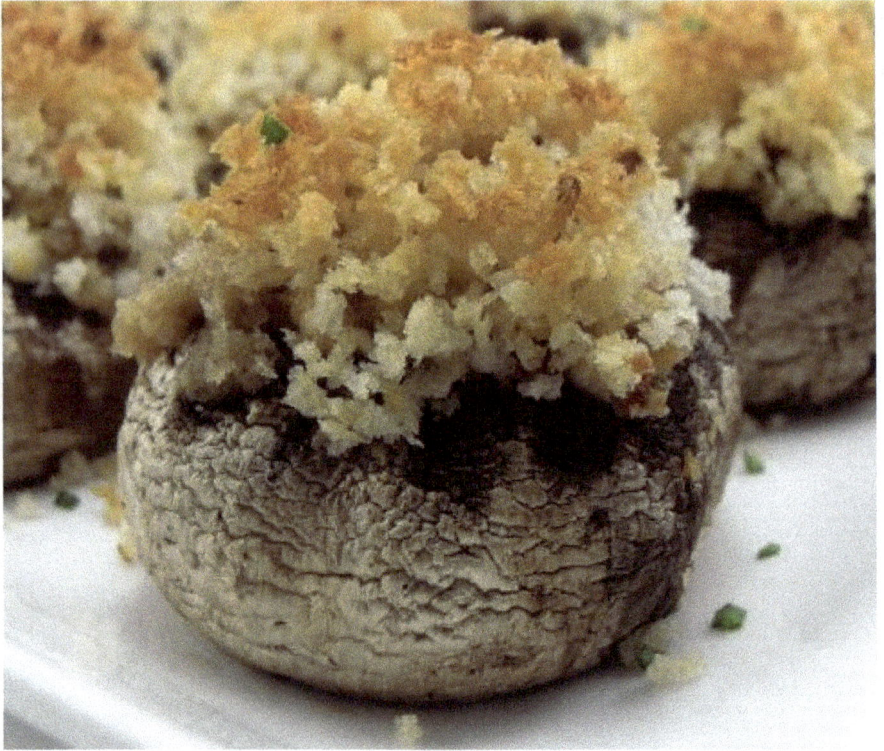

Tomato Sandwiches with Feta and Pesto

Preparation Time: 60 min

Servings: 2

Nutrition Values: Calories: 41; Carbs: 5g; Fat: 4g; Protein: 2g

Ingredients

- 1 heirloom tomato

- 1 -4- ozblock Feta cheese

- 1 small red onion, thinly sliced

- 1 clove garlic

- Salt to taste

- 2 tsp + ¼ cup olive oil

- 1 ½ tbsp toasted pine nuts

- ¼ cup chopped parsley

- ¼ cup grated Parmesan cheese

- ¼ cup chopped basil

Directions

1. Add basil, pine nuts, garlic and salt to a food processor. Process while adding the ¼ cup of olive oil slowly. Once the oil is finished, pour the basil pesto into a bowl and refrigerate for 30 minutes. Preheat the Air fryer to 390 F.

2. Slice the feta cheese and tomato into ½ inch circular slices. Use a kitchen towel to pat the tomatoes dry. Remove the pesto from the fridge and use a tablespoon to spread some pesto on each slice of tomato. Top with a slice of feta cheese. Add the onion and remaining olive oil in a bowl and toss. Spoon on top of feta cheese.

3. Place the tomato in the fryer's basket and cook for 12 minutes. Remove to a serving platter, sprinkle lightly with salt and top with the remaining pesto. Serve with a side of rice or lean meat.

Italian style Tofu

Preparation time: 30 min

Servings: 2

Nutrition Values: Calories: 87; Carbs: 3.4g;
Fat: 4.4g; Protein: 10g

Ingredients

- 6 oz extra firm tofu
- pepper to season
- 1 tbsp vegetable broth
- 1 tbsp soy sauce
- ⅓ tsp dried oregano
- ⅓ tsp garlic powder
- ⅓ tsp dried basil
- ⅓ tsp onion powder

Directions

1. Place the tofu on a cutting board, and cut it into 3 lengthwise slices with a knife. Line a side of the cutting board with paper towels, place the tofu on it and cover with paper towel. Use your hands to press the tofu

gently until as much liquid has been extracted from it.

2. Remove the paper towels and use a knife to chop the tofu into 8 cubes; set aside. In another bowl, add the soy sauce, vegetable broth, oregano, basil, garlic powder, onion powder, and black pepper; mix well with a spoon.

3. Pour the spice mixture on the tofu, stir the tofu until well coated; set aside to marinate for 10 minutes. Preheat the Air Fryer to 390 F, and arrange the tofu in the fryer's basket, in a single layer; cook for 10 minutes, flipping it at the 6-minute mark. Remove to a plate and serve with green salad.

Two-Cheese Vegetable Frittata

Preparation Time: 35 min

Servings: 2

Nutrition Values: Calories: 203; Carbs: 9.3g; Fat: 15.2g; Protein: 6.4g

Ingredients

- 1 cup baby spinach
- ⅓ cup sliced mushrooms
- 1 large zucchini, sliced with a 1-inch thickness
- 1 small red onion, sliced
- ¼ cup chopped chives
- ¼ lb asparagus, trimmed and sliced thinly
- 2 tsp olive oil
- 4 eggs, cracked into a bowl
- ⅓ cup milk
- Salt and pepper to taste
- ⅓ cup grated Cheddar cheese

- ⅓ cup crumbled Feta cheese

Directions

1. Preheat the Air Fryer to 320 F and line a 6 x 6 inches baking dish with parchment paper; set aside. In the egg bowl, add milk, salt, and pepper; beat evenly. Place a skillet over medium heat on a stove top, and heat olive oil.

2. Add the asparagus, zucchini, onion, mushrooms, and baby spinach; stir-fry for 5 minutes. Pour the veggies into the baking dish and top with the egg mixture. Sprinkle feta and cheddar cheese over and place in the Air Fryer.

3. Cook for 15 minutes. Remove the baking dish and garnish with fresh chives.

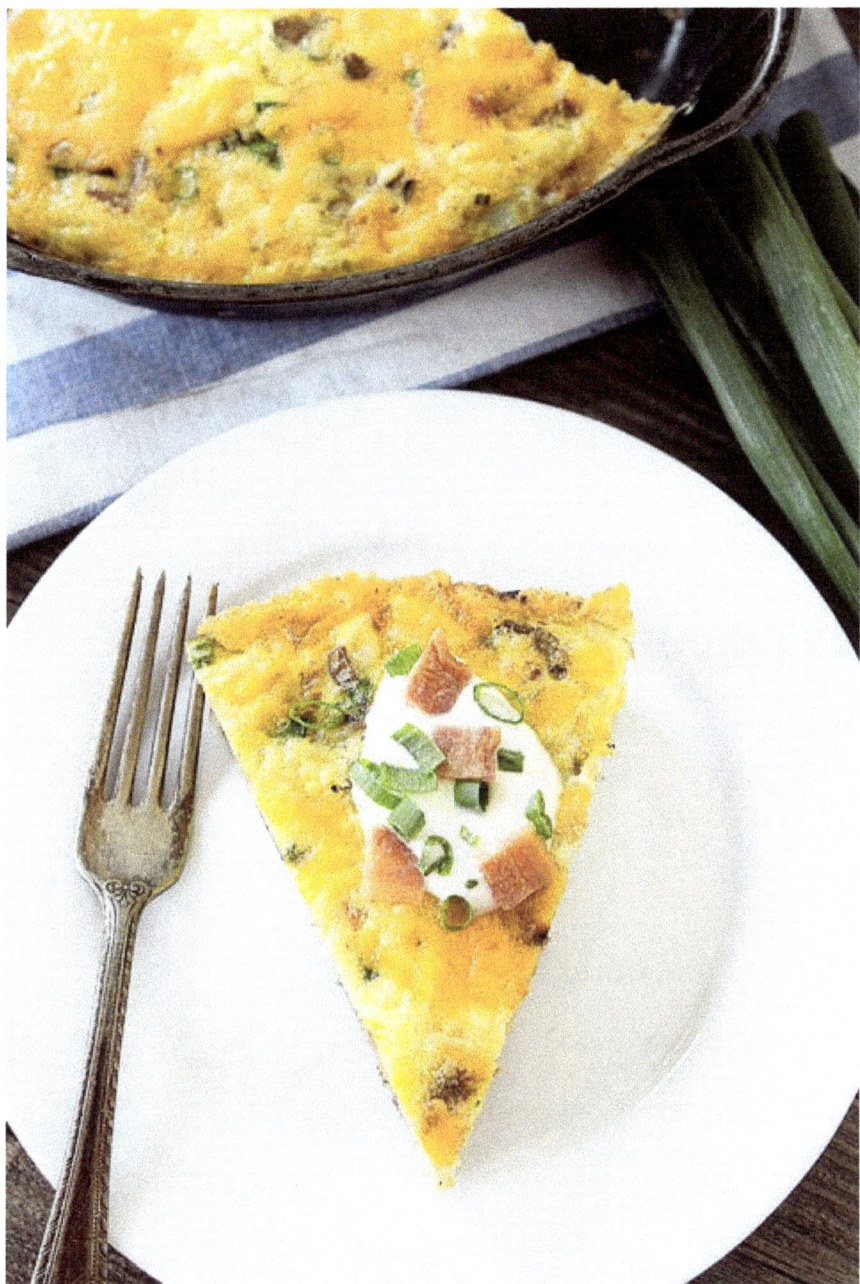